Happy Guide to a Greener You

A guide to a better lifestyle

Susana Aldanondo

ISBN-13:
978-1986902229

ISBN-10:
1986902226

TABLE OF CONTENTS

-Break the Cycle

-No debit

-Decluttering

-The Equation

-Children Turning Green

-Be informed

-World Organizations

-Turning Green and Staying Green

Inspirational quotes and a space to write are included.

Introduction

Happy Guide to a Greener You will guide you to make better decisions about what matters in life, about what you need to sustain a healthy lifestyle, and about thinking what trash really means. Is it something we create? Is it something we buy?

Is   ***it***   ***a***   ***lifestyle?***

Trash is by definition: junk, litter, waste. Have you ever worried about how we all seem to be contributing to a plastic, chemical, trash filled world? From the moment you wake up to the time you set your head on your pillow at night, all the "in between" moments of decisions you've made have played a role in the kind of world you want for yourself and future generations.

It's not that just one more "cup'o joe" from the trendy coffee shop doesn't count, it does, it really does count, and add up to the grey, dirty, tree-less, air polluted, plastic filled, life for all of us, and all who are yet to be born into this world. Making a change is urgent. It is the right thing to do.

The only thing we can all do to make a change, to stop the direction of the wasteland effect that the world is headed to, is to commit to making a change in our lifestyle. As a mother, as a human being, I have often pondered on all of the above and more. It's not easy to break free of learned behaviors, learned habits and commodities.

We, as humans, must take a step in the right direction. That direction is to be found as we look in the opposite direction of all those learned behaviors.

Throw them out the window! Start anew! Think about recycling: how is recycling being abused into the new norm? Recycle your thoughts, not things. And by this I don't mean you should not make the meaningful attempt to recycle that which you may otherwise throw away, no. All I mean is: don't indulge in the prospect of wasteful purchases because you can later recycle those purchases. Use your life as the recycling bin *where* *waste* *stops.* Think of how so many of the traditions we follow started and why they started. Ask yourself if teaching those same traditions to future generations will be a step in the direction our planet needs. If you think you're ready to make the change, I invite you to read on.

THE WASTEFUL INDUSTRY

Think about what moves the world.
If you thought money: you got it right.
The paper industry is a $2.6 billion-dollar industry.

Paper wrapping and decorations account for about half
of the approximate 85 million tons of paper products
Americans consume each year. Wrapping paper and
shopping bags account for around 4 million tons of trash
produced in the U.S.

The fact is, we are wasting trees, the very source of clean
air, shade, and source of life, to wrap gifts.
To create waste.
According to the Clean Air Council, in the United States,
"a total of an additional 5 million tons of waste is
produced over the Christmas gift giving period."
This amounts to 30 million trees cut down just so that we
can wrap gifts, according to Tree Hugger.
We are by this, working against the environment. Trees
are the source of air, they are the lungs of your block,
city, state, country and our earth.

Our bodies need clean air to breath.

Trees act as a filter to renew the air we breathe.

According to research, poor air quality can contribute to
chronic disease such as "asthma and cardiovascular
disease."

There is so much information that we each need to
become aware of to make better choices for our
environment and for ourselves.

Think about all the money the paper industry alone
makes from our gift giving traditions.

Think about how absurd this is, we pay expensive prices
to buy wrapping paper and paper decorations for gifts,
which accounts for 30 million trees being cut down,
which accounts for 4 million tons of waste regularly and
5 million tons of waste during our holiday season! for
the reason of: concealing an object for a few seconds,
until its wrapping paper is torn and discarded. It's a
socially approved behavior, not doing so would be out of
the ordinary, out of the box, a weird thing to do.

And we are all responsible.

Whatever you do, your children are
learning to do as well, the same goes for gift wrapping
traditions. It's a never-ending cycle of waste.

Wasted trees, for a few seconds of concealing an item, then into the waste basket!

And please, don't try to do the world a favor by reducing waste by burning the used gift wraps, as most of these contain metals and chemicals that when burnt can produce gases that are hazardous to your health.

We must learn about where the traditions we use so gallantly and so innately come from.

Gift wrapping tradition is just one of the many traditions we follow blindly without knowing why and what effect it has on the environment and what we are teaching our little ones.

It doesn't stop there, think about the cardboard box the gift was attached to, and how the pallets that brought all those boxes to the store were wrapped in plastic. More waste right there. For every pound of wrapping paper there are several pounds of cardboard, blister packs and twist tags.
There is so much waste that surrounds a single gift.
And all this information does not tackle the rest of the waste involved in our celebratory traditions, think of all the wasteful plastic involved in goodie bags, invitations,

greeting cards, disposable plates and cups, forks and spoons.

Open your cupboards, look around your home, and the list goes on.

It all adds to the deforestation of our world, and the creation of endless waste.

Let's be informed and break the cycle. That's what turning green, it's about a journey, a lifestyle, a new way to make decisions, a new frame of mind, an acquired trait that we identify with. When you make the decision to turn green, your life will take a turn for the better, setting the right example for your children, your friends, your neighbors, the owner of the store you purchase food items from, your school, your students, your fellow subway commuters, etc.

Turning Green is making the decision to make changes to your lifestyle, regardless of traditions, learned behaviors and what we're so used to that has become our norm and we do automatically. Living a greener life means you make a shift in the way you decide how to live your life, realizing you have an impact on your own life,

others' lives, and the world near and far.
Because we should all be trying to a achieve a greener
version of ourselves..

"The goal in life is to make your heartbeat match the beat of the universe, to match your nature with Nature."
~Joseph Campbell

Make a list of things you want to do that can bring you closer to nature:

GIFT WRAPPING TRADITIONS

The tradition of gift wrapping has been around for ages, dating back to ancient China. It can also be found in the Japanese culture, although it is less common nowadays as the Japanese are more conscientious and have returned to the use of the *furoshiki,* a cloth wrapping tradition.

So how did the Western world become so "wrapped up"? The Victorian elite used to conceal gifts with elaborate paper. By the 20th century the practice was echoed by a more practical gift wrapping service provided by stores.

In the year 1917, two brothers Joyce and Rollie Hall, who owned a stationary store, were having a phenomenal holiday season at their store, in fact so phenomenal that they ran out of the traditional tissue like wrapping paper.

Digging through their inventory, they found French paper that was used as lining for envelopes. That accidental decision to use that paper and put it up for sale in their store, would shape our

traditions, and shape our world as we know it. So seeing
all the waste in the trash cans after Christmas mornings,
thank the Hall brothers. And thank everyone else who
are following the Hall brothers' business oriented mind
frame for the use of paper, without even knowing why
we need to wrap gifts to begin with.
But don't let those two brothers and the billion-dollar
paper industry make up your mind on what traditions to
follow.

Let the trees, air, water, earth and future generations be
the source of inspiration to break free and find new,
better and sustainable traditions.

The world has evolved in so many ways, however, the
billion dollar industries keep the world stuck in the year
1917. The world has other needs, we are better informed
and most of us want to contribute to the world in a
positive way. We wish to help our environment, and we
want to make better choices. Make the decision to find
new, more sustainable traditions then. Goodbye year
1917, we care about the world.

"And forget not that the earth delights to feel your bare feet, and the wind longs to play with your hair."~Khalil Gibran

Do you give yourself opportunities to enjoy the outdoors? Do you feel alive in the world? Do something this week that will remind you of how you belong to the earth and the earth belongs to you:

HISTORY OF THE DISPOSABLE SHOPPING BAG

Oh all those plastic bags at the supermarket!, all those plastic bags I see floating like kites, propelled by winds!. Oh all those plastic bags found in trash cans, in our rivers, and oceans, polluting habitats and causing irreparable harm!. Oh, how I think about the 400 years each one of those bags will take to decompose. I feel sadness, at the sight of each plastic bag. In the year 2005, I took a pledge not to use anymore plastic bags. I purchased canvas totes and bags. I am proud of it, and wish I'd see more people doing so, if not all.

How did the disposable shopping bag come to be?

Prior to the 1850's, people shopped in the city markets and carried their groceries home in carts or in canvas bags.
By 1852, a school teacher named France's Wolle, invented the first machine to make paper bags and patented it.
In 1912, a grocery store owner in Minnesota named Walter Deubener, used chords to reinforce paper bags and add handles so that his customers could comfortably

carry any purchased items and thus, increase sales.
The bags became known as *"Deubener Shopping Bags"*
and by 1915, he had sold over a million
bags. His bags became the standard for of bag available
at stores.

Then by the 1960's Swedish Sten Gustaf Thulin
developed the thin lightweight and cost efficient plastic
bags. By 1975, the plastic bag started to be the norm for
most stores because of its affordability.

We now know what a pollutant the plastic bag is, and
countries such as Germany, South Africa, Australia,
Belgium, Turkey, Sweden, Chile, Bangladesh, India,
Ireland, Italy, among others, have banned plastic bags
according to Surfrider.org

Sadly, except for Chile where the use of plastic bags is
banned, the use of plastic bags is at large in Central and
the rest of South America.

In the United States of America, only the states of
California and Hawaii have banned the use of plastic bags.

The plastic industry thrives on, making it a multi-billion-
dollar Industry and making clear strides toward
continuing to pollute the planet. The question remains to

18

be answered by each and every one of us: at what cost? Some become rich and direct the world's catastrophic future. Our oceans are suffering, there is plastic waste ending up in our streets, rivers and oceans, killing birds and marine life, polluting our waters and breaking down the health of our ecosystems. Plastics don't break down, most won't biodegrade. It takes 400 years for a single lightweight plastic bag to disappear.

So, think about it. The change is urgent, it must happen now, you are an important decision maker and difference maker to the world, so is your next-door neighbor, so is the owner and cashier of the supermarket where you shop, so is your employer. Everyone counts. Everyone is a contributor.

You must decide if you'll be a contributor to the waste catastrophe or if you'll be a part of the solution. I want to be part of the solution. If you're still reading this book, I know you too want to be a part of the solution. I know there are still many people out there making poor decisions, some doing so carelessly, but some doing so because they lack the information they need to give this some thought and a chance.

What energy are you creating within you and for those around you? Are you a propeller of peaceful empathy and understanding? Are you creating a path to a better world?

BACKGROUND: GREEN

We all come from somewhere. Our backgrounds play an important role in how we see the world, what we value most, how we treasure memories, how we celebrate, how we live. Traditions, how we relate to our community, how we see the environment, has a lot to do with how and where we grew up and the traditions we were given to hold as ours. You will read more about traditions in this book, and I want to let you know that this book is not about criticizing traditions nor not respecting them, I am an advocate of diversity and respect. I advocate to the right we each have as human beings and inhabitants of this planet to ensure that we align with those traditions when it comes to our lives and the environment. Perhaps making small changes to some traditions we hold dear will help so as you practice and honor your traditions, you also honor your humanity and your beliefs about being environmentally friendly. That's what my family and I have done as we choose to celebrate Christmas with an open mind about what we want it to be about.

This book portrays my experience, loaded with memories of my childhood growing up in a middle-class family household.

As I look back into my childhood I can grasp the sense of a naturally green, environmentally friendly lifestyle. Accidentally, as a given, since that was the case for most people back then.

My childhood memories consist of lots of play time outside, fond memories of home-cooked meals, a beautifully decorated dinner table, clothed with tablecloths made and crocheted by my grandmother, real glass cups, real porcelain tea cups, real porcelain plates to serve snacks and foods. Cloth napkins. Silverware.

I remember receiving gifts during my birthday parties, but I do not remember my parents taking out bags with the waste product each gift had created. Christmas was another occasion of modesty.

No paper goods nor paper decorations. Cloth table cloths and porcelain plates and bowls would be set on the dinner table. Our finances didn't allow splurging in gifts, yet, I don't remember a single Christmas when I complained. I was happy, I was content even the year I got a knitted headband as a gift. It was *the* headband I wanted. It was pink, with a bow on top. I loved it. I was around nine years old at the time, and I remember combing my hair and positioning the bow in a way that would look chic. Someone took a picture of me wearing that headband, and I still have the picture, but what strikes me most, is the simplicity of the thought of being content with a single, most wanted, most wished for, chic, headband.

I have fond loving memories that did not require materialistic means to be engraved in my soul forever, on the contrary, the feeling of everything being so "real" so not "disposable" remains in me and fills me with joy, because life takes on a different look when we don't make it as disposable as the industry wants us to.

My mother's cooking was real, all the porcelain platters spread out over the dinner table, showcasing her most delicious foods, for birthday parties, the holiday season, and her daily cooking, it was just so real. My memories aren't disposable, they are engraved in my heart, her hands cooking, her baking, her dedication, they were all worth the most exquisite porcelain diner set.

Memories seem more real, prettier, and more special.

I realize today's world and all that it demands from each of us may not allow for us to think we have the time for all those reusable moments. But I also know that this never ending cycle of disposable items and memory making, easy and get it done fast ways are not sustainable. I know the disposable cycle in which we seem to have been sucked into may make cleaning up faster, easier, we all have such busy lives to run, for sure, but it doesn't take so much longer to wash, and put certain things away, instead of just throwing cups and plates away. I haven't used any disposable cups, plates or even spoons and forks at my children's birthday parties. We don't use paper plates at home. We don't even use paper towels. We don't use paper napkins. The list goes on. It isn't easy at times, making those changes does require effort, and I don't question those who do use all those disposable items because believe me, I know how difficult it is to do everything we have to do, particularly families with children! I take my hat off for all working, non-working mothers and fathers! We do so much! But, as part of the mission of this book I am here to encourage you! Encourage you not only for all that you do, but to try the changes you might think are too difficult or that would place even more loads of work on your shoulders. I can relate. I here ask you to try it in small steps. Breaking down the daunting task of living a greener life can help you make the change a smooth transition. It can help you realize that it's really more about creating new habits, it might take some extra time at first, but then you'll realize that it all becomes a part of how do things.

Those small changes, those tiny steps you take, turn out to be part of a new set of routines and ways in which you run your daily errands and do your daily tasks.

"You cannot go through a single day without having an impact on the world around you. What you do makes a difference. And you have to decide what kind of difference you want to make." ~Jane Goodall

Write about how you impact the world around you: your family, your block, your city. How do you think you can be an example of change?

DO'S & DON'T'S

So, here's a list of the "Don'ts" on the left side followed by the the "Do's" on the right side.

-No paper towel – Cleaning reusable towels.

-No paper plates – Porcelain/ceramic dish set

-No plastic/paper cups – Glass jam jars we recycle to use as cups.

-No plastic utensils – silverware and bamboo forks, spoons and knives.

-No baby wipes – cloth baby wipes we wash and reuse

-No feminine pads – homemade cloth pads

-No shampoo related waste – we make our own

-No toothpaste related waste – we make our own

-No laundry detergent waste – we make our own

-No plastic grocery bags – we use canvas grocery bags

-No plastic produce bags – we used cloth reusable produce bags.

-No fruit/veggie packaging – we buy lose fruit and vegetables.

-No cereal/legume packaging – we buy bulk at the organic store.

-No plastic water bottles – we always bring our own water in reusable water bottles.

-No floor wipes/cleaning sheets – we always mop with the traditional kind of mop.

-No click to shop – Shop local

-No gift wrapping – we only wrap in fabric or reusable bags

-No Christmas Tree cutting, we have a couple of evergreens in front of our place which we decorate and light. You can purchase a small tree to keep in your apartment, and have it for years, if it gets too big you could either plant it outside or donate it to your community garden or local park.

-No Christmas gift wrapping – we leave fabric bags by the tree so Santa, who also cares about the earth, can put any gifts inside. That is, if you believe in Santa!

Expanding this list is one of my set goals for life. Start your list today. Set clear goals.

Create a list of changes you can implement around your household. List the items you usually purchase and what you can replace them with as a greener alternative:

TRADITIONS

Tradition is, by definition, the transmission of customs or beliefs from generation to generation.

What a great responsibility weighing on the shoulders of the generation giving passing traditions on to the next generation. I want to highlight that I am aware that not all traditions create waste, nor do I want by writing about this to shame nor create any hostile feelings toward the traditions I mention, nor none that you as a reader may hold dear. I love diversity, different cultures, there is so much to learn from each culture, this is something that I honor and respect: diversity and culture, people's backgrounds and beliefs.

Traditions, just like habits, good or bad, will be transmitted to our youngsters. Wrapping gifts with paper wrap, is a tradition that has basically been imposed onto our generation. It seems unstoppable as so many other things do. The wasteful purchases made so that we'll present someone a gift on certain occasions, instead of giving our loved ones the gift of our time and attention, the gift of doing something they truly love or hope to do, or making such a gift. None of that seems to be the norm.

Wasteful presentations through décor and the excitement of concealing an item for a few moments before it is revealed upon the exaltation of ripping papers and opening paper bags have replaced the true meanings of the occasions we celebrate this modern life.

Do you agree? Do you agree with at least some of what you've read so far? Even if you agree on some of the points I've described, you can start on your journey of change. Your grain of sand does count. As does mine, and my children's, and one day their children's. We must take the first step. We must act as role models in this sense as well. Because we are. We are being watched. We are being admired.

We are creating memories, and traditions, and habits. Let them be good ones, healthy ones, positive ones. Let us take responsibility for decades of carelessness. Decades of waste. Decades of tons of waste. Let us take responsibility and not contribute to the billion-dollar paper and plastic industries.

Let's reduce waste. Let's reuse items. Let's celebrate without wasting precious resources. Let's live without contributing to the death of our planet.

"It is not enough to be busy. So are the ants. The question is: what are you busy about?"~Henry David Thoreau

Write about what traditions you are willing to give up in order to live a greener better life:

TINY STEPS

Making a change from the lifestyle that our society promotes as the norm isn't easy. Not only has society been telling us certain things are the thing to do, the way to celebrate, and what's expected, but mostly we get all that information from our parents and peers as well. So taking on the task to become more environmentally friendly isn't a particularly easy subject you can tackle in one step. The fact that you thought about this and picked this book to read is testimony that you're headed in the right direction of change.

So many of the learned and acceptable norms that are such a pollutant to our world have been absorbed and tattooed onto our beings, our lifestyle, our day to day living. How do we untangle the intangible? How to undo all that has been written on our "to do" list of things we are to do?

For instance, your employer is hosting a holiday party and everyone is asked to bring a gift for someone in the office, such as the Secret Santa usually a popular way to give without each person having to buy a gift for each and every one at the office, so yes, suppose it's that time of the year again, and you must buy a gift for one of your colleagues. Got the gift. Now the norm is: get gift wrap, tissue paper, a paper bag, a card. How would you change that process if you were to live a green life?

See, it's not just carrying your reusable bag to the grocery store that makes you a "green" person, it's actually much more than just your trip to the store that plays a role in how "green" your impact on the world will or will not be.

So yes, baby steps, but with the "greener" big picture in mind.

If you were one of those people who always get a plastic bag at the store, the supermarket, the pharmacy, the deli, but you started carrying your own reusable bags now and you are feeling great and feeling you are making a difference, you are walking in the right direction. My thought about this is, "keep walking". Don't stop at the exhilaration of knowing you are using less plastic. Keep making small changes to your routines, don't let your reusable bag use be the only step you take. You are the only person who knows exactly what you need and how you live your life on a day to day basis. You're the only person who knows that drinking your coffee on the subway or train may be the only way you can get a warm drink during the mornings. The world tells us to rush, run, hurry, work schedules sometimes force us to wake up very early, or end our work day very late. Each person's world, needs and demands are different and unique. You will know what step to take next. You will be the only person to decide when it will be your turn to start making the change the world needs. I hope it won't take you too long. Everyone's effort is valuable and can make a positive impact felt on the world around us and in each other. We are society.

Make the next change one that you, your needs and life's demands can handle. All change seems difficult at first, until we think about how possible it is for us to make the change.

Keep walking, even if they are baby steps, they move us all in the right direction.

Some baby steps you may want to consider:

-First and foremost: carry your own reusable water bottle. Don't buy bottled water as much as possible.

-Buy the milk that comes in the vintage- like glass bottles. Return to the store when finished, and there is no waste involved!

-Buy bulk whenever possible. A local organic store in our city carries bulk laundry detergent, softener, and dish soap. You bring your own bottle or container and buy those items bulk. Your clean clothes, and dishes, no longer create all that plastic and cardboard waste.

-As much as possible, buy local. Not only will you benefit all the local shops in your community, but you'll be supporting a way to shop that creates less waste. Hitting "click" from any device is easy, but think of all the fuel and cardboard boxes a purchase can be responsible for.

-Stop buying coffee. Get a reusable mug with a lid and make your own coffee at home before you leave for work. If possible, make your own coffee at work too, using that same mug or another one you can leave at work.

-Don't buy anymore paper gift wrap, paper bags, nor tissue paper. Instead, buy some fabric from your local fabric store, and sew the edges to make the neat, and apply some Velcro to the sides. If you're not the crafty type, there are several fabric wrapping options for sale online, and a few clicks can revolutionize the way you give gifts forever. A really nice option for lager gifts is just getting a few nice pillow cases and repurposing them to use in the art of "gift giving". Another option, is getting the canvas like reusable shopping bag from your local .99 cent store and using those.

One thing you can do is ask the person you're giving the gift to, to return the fabric wrap or bag, so you won't be having to purchase those repeatedly.

-Christmas. For Christmas, you can do the same as previously discussed about any other gift. Purchase canvas like totes, you might find the kind that are made Christmas themed fabric, or you could make your own with fabrics you like. You could also buy plain canvas bags.

We do this every year, we place our reusable gift bags by the tree and then when Santa comes along, he just places the gifts in the bags. No gift-wrapping waste from us during the holiday season.

-Cotton dish cloths are perfect everyday napkins, without all the waste that paper towels or paper napkins produce. Switch to those! Any .99 cent store has them and they are super affordable.

-Carry your own fork and spoon and fabric napkin in your purse or bag.

-Cotton cleaning towels. Also, very affordable and available at most .99 cent stores.

No paper towels needed when you have these available. You can clean up any mess and then toss them in the laundry hamper. Wash and reuse.

-Of course, carry your own shopping bags in your purse or car. Depending on the size of your family, carry as many as you'll need on any trip to the supermarket. Don't forget to let the cashier know you have your own bags. Sometimes they're too quick and they start to bag items before you can remember to mention your bags.

-If you have little ones, tell them why doing what you do- such as bringing your own bag, or buying bulk, is important. Reusing seems to always create waste, using items that don't generate waste is key.

Write about what things matter to you the most, and what moves you to take steps to make changes in your lifestyle:

HISTORY OF THE DISPOSABLE CUP

The option to the communal cup, traced back to the 20th century, when temperance activists dotted cities with water fountains and traveled from city to city offering water as an alternative to beer and liquor, and offered the water served in a communal cup. During the same time frame, there was more awareness of health concerns and this concern led a Boston based lawyer and inventor to invent the paper cup, envisioning the need to prevent disease, and promote a healthier option to the communal cup. He first named his invention the Health Kup, but later changed the name to Dixie Rolls.

Before WWI, the fix and reuse way of life was the norm. Little was discarded. So, the idea didn't quite catch on. In 1918, when thousands got sick with a flu epidemic, the idea of the healthier disposable cup was given a second chance, a new era begun. Dixie cups were used to drink water. A disposable cup to drink hot beverages was yet to be developed. Some inventors invented paper cups with handles, to be able to carry hot beverages, in an effort to mimic mugs. It wasn't until the 1960's that reusable cups designed to hold hot drinks hit the streets. In 1963, a

Czech immigrant named Leslie Buck designed the "Anthora" cup for a coffee shop in Connecticut, and it became, as The New York Times called it in 1995, "the most successful cup in history."

In 1964, 7-Eleven was the first store to sell "on the go" coffee. The rest is history.

"Unless someone like you cares a whole awful lot, nothing is going to get better, it's not" ~Dr. Seuss

Write about what you'll do today to stop the use of disposable cups, plastic water bottles and the like:

WHY HISTORY

As I usually tell my children: history is so important. It tells us about our country, other countries, cultures, important events, and important places which help us understand the city, state, and world we live in.

History answers some of the "why's" and "when's" that shape our society.

It's crucial to learn the "why's" and "when's" of the available choices. Why are certain things a given in our daily interactions? Why are things that hurt the overall health of our planet still available? Why am I using items or services that may contribute to the high levels of waste and pollution our world has sunk into?

Why does an invention that served a purpose in the year 1917, or in the 1960's but creates a huge problem for the world today and for generations to come, still have such an influence on the way we live today? Why hasn't that idea evolved? Why don't politicians and elected government officials help propel those changes? And if that's the case, why don't we each, with our free will power make a difference for the better?

Questions need answers. Decisions need questions. History can help provide some answers to those questions so we may make better, more educated decisions. Our children and our planet desperately need us to make informed decisions.

Will you be drinking coffee in disposable cups because a Boston lawyer invented a kind of disposable cup in his efforts to stop people from sharing a cup everyone in town used to get a drink of water? Will you continue to walk into your local coffee shop or chain restaurant and purchase a cup of coffee in a disposable cup because a store decided to start selling coffee on the go using that disposable mentality of the 1960's?

Or will you step up to the year we all live in, knowing what we now know, and make the necessary changes to stop the disposable madness the world has turned into?

I'm not saying not to buy a cup of coffee at your local coffee shop, if that's part of your routine, no, all I'm saying is: bring your own mug.

We're not living in the 60's- we've evolved. And in the process, we've trashed the planet with coffee cups, lids, water bottles, and endless plastics and cardboard items. Let's really, truly evolve, because to evolve means to make progress. Let's make progress in the little things that add up to big things. Coffee cups are one of those things.

Evolve using real, reusable options.

Let's make progress and end the use of disposable coffee cups.

Think back to your childhood days and think of how certain memories made an impact on how you make decisions today, did you rush out of your home without having breakfast at the dinner table? Did you drink out of plastic bottles? Make the list:

BREAK THE CYCLE

Life can be expensive, the more we seem to want and need, the more items you will want to acquire, the more money you will have to designate to obtain those items, the longer hours you will need to work to be able to afford those items. The more items you have, add up and you may find yourself having to give up closet space to store items. You may find yourself hiring a storage unit, creating an additional expense, having to spend yet more time working, and caring for those things, and the cycle continues.

Getting you farther away from the quality time you and your loved ones want and deserve. For what? Things?

Is it really worth it? Are material things really worth minutes and hours of your life? Because that's what it comes down to. You trade hours of your life to earn money, and in turn, you spend money on things. And those things put you to work too.

It's time to realize what you value in life. Things? Or the people you love? The activities you love? Do you have time to spend with your loved ones? Do you have time to

do the things you love? Are you working your life away?
The result: a less fulfilled, tired, stress, overworked,
frustrated, more isolated you. You are an easier prey to
all those advertisements, an easier prey to all those stores
flashing sales before your eyes.

The less you have, the less money you spend on things.
The less time you will have to work to get things.
There will be no need to pay for a storage unit, your closet
will be good to store the things you do need and wear.
You will find things more easily. You will have time to
spend with loved ones and do activities you like. The
result: a more fulfilled, happier you.

So I say yes, less is more. To learn this, we must break
the cycle.

Look around your house, your closet, start seeing the items you own and ask what the purpose of the items that make you –pause to think- is:

NO DEBIT-NO CREDIT CARDS

Stop buying things just because they are on sale. They may be on sale, yes, they may even be a good buy, but the real question to ask yourself before you go to a store and make a purchase is: do I need this? You may feel like you do need it, of course, the sale price, all the perks the item offers, or how lovely it looks on you or on the mannequin. But "do you need it? Or does the store need you to spend your money, so the sale is the hook they use to reel you into the store?

Walk away. Give it a 48 hour wait period. Wait it out. Waiting to decide on whether you need an item can work wonders. If you really do need the item, for sure do buy it, but not before the 48 hour wait it out period is up. Most of the time you will realize you didn't really need or want the item, in fact, you already have a similar shirt or the pants you have will do, or if the item is an appliance, maybe there isn't an immediate need for it. The money the store wanted you to waste, is still in your pocket, or bank account.

Waiting is a winner on shopping matters.

It will save you money, space and longer working hours.

Another strategy is to leave your ATM card at home. Carry cash for your commute and weekly needs, but leave the ATM card at home. By doing this, we could save money, it really does work. It is so easy and tempting to swipe your card and make a purchase, but it is a whole different scenario when you carry cash, for when your cash is limited, so is your purchasing power, and waiting to decide on a purchase is a must.

Use the money you save wisely. If you have credit card debt, use the money you save in all the items you didn't buy to pay for those debts. Use your money wisely. Put your money to work toward the kind of life you seek. It all seems to add up to move your life in the direction of a less cluttered, less wasteful life, in its full sense.

Less waste = Less stuff = More space = More room to live = More time to dedicate to your life = A happier you with a more meaningful life. An added plus: you will also have more available money, unspent on "stuff" which will open new possibilities for saving, paying off debt,

Write some thoughts on what you believe you need less of and what you need more of in your life:

DECLUTTERING

Agrrrrrr!- is what I feel when I look around and see clothes, boxes, books, decorations, furniture, toys, and closets filled with more of the already mentioned, among other things.

Where to start? How to start?

So many things seem to interrupt the healthy smooth flow you envision for your home or office space. This is part of the wasteful mind frame that has been installed in you and which you are trying to change, as you learn about the choices you've made when making purchases, and as you learn to take tiny steps, as you honor the "48 hour wait period" before making a purchase, as you take in the thought that less is more.

I see it in my children, they had so many toys, so many that about two hours per day would be dedicated to putting those toys away. Toys they had taken out, but not really played with. They had so many options to choose from and would end up just leaving the toys all over the place without really making any use of any of them. So I put away most toys, each hand-picked five toys they really loved and wanted to play with. The rest were stored away. They played with those toys. They had less options but the quality of their interactions with those options got better and meaningful. Clean up time was reduced to 10 minutes.

My rule is: keep what you love. Keep only what will bring happiness and a positive outlook. Retire the rest.

In the case of children's items, involve them in this process, and don't throw away their things. Store them away, and then one day you can have them "exchange toys" from the storage boxes. Stop buying toys, unless they will contribute to the health, and education of your child. But it's important that you respect their choices and feelings, make the list of toys to be kept longer to accommodate their needs and their feelings.

Any other items:

Make signs to designate areas to help you decide. One of them will be labeled as "Keep", the next will be labeled "Maybe" and the next will be labeled "Give away-Donate".

As you look through the room, make sure you first place the items you are sure about throwing out or donating.

How will you decide? Well, think and ask yourself if the item serves or will serve a purpose that will contribute to your life in any way? If the answer is no: give it away. And make a point not to replace the item. Write down the item on the "Give-away-Donate" list.

Anything you need to think about, consult or reconsider, put in the "Maybe" pile.

Any items that help you in your daily routine, which you look forward to using, wearing, or that may have a purpose for the future, place in the keep file.

Reconsider the "Maybe" and "Keep" piles. Got through all items and try to find some more items that might not serve any purpose other than to clutter your home or office space. Ask yourself: if I store this item away, will I need it and must look for it? If the answer is "no", then move the item to the "Give-away-Donate" pile. If the answer is "yes", then move the item to the "Keep" pile.

When did acquiring "stuff" replace the sense of happiness and fulfillment? How did the two become a part of a same thought? Perhaps it's a personal question we each should ask ourselves.

The answer to that question may be found deep in memories of our childhood, our understanding of happiness may be tainted by the need to have things, erroneously, but we might make that connection. Perhaps for others, "stuff", fills a hole in their lives for the lack of close family ties, or friendships. The answer may be found in the kind of human experience we find in our surroundings. Do we live in a city that constantly tells us that if we buy "stuff" we'll finally feel happy? Are we being told that we need stuff to be happy, better looking, and enjoy life. Quote me on this, as this may have the opposite effect on your life. Things won't buy you happiness. They will most likely buy you debt and long hours at work for you instead. You will enjoy life with less money available in your bank account, left for leisure, or for savings. But having less, sometimes won't fix whatever inner search you must go through in your life, my hope is that this guide and these steps will help you in your quest to get to feel more joy and less stress in your life. Doing so is a journey, really, and I hope this guide will help you in your journey, and as you go through life I also hope that the changes you can make, such as the ones I've written about here can help you feel more connected to nature and the environment around you, and in feeling more connected you may realize that it really does come full circle to impact your life with a positive feeling. The more connected we are to our environment and to nature, the more we can live a better life, fix the things that need fixing in our lives and make decisions that align with what you want for your life. So, in if you think about it, turning green can help the environment but also, and equally as important, can help you feel more aligned with the world, can help you become more aware of the things you need and don't need to achieve joy, peace, and which lead to a better life.

"When one tugs at a single thing in nature, he finds it attached to the rest of the world "~John Muir

Think about and make a list of items you pledge not to buy anymore, since they don't have a useful purpose in your life:

THE EQUATION

As a rule of thumb, remember: when things stop adding up in your life, it's time to start subtracting.

Subtract things, money spent, plastic, cardboard, packages, plastic water bottles, disposable items, disposable coffee cups, disposable diapers, disposable wipes, disposable napkins, and disposable paper towels, disposable utensils, disposable cups, disposable tablecloths, anything disposable that turns into waste. Waste that will end up in landfills, waste that will be subtracted from your bank account, waste that will mean millions of trees subtracted from the earth, waste that will translate into health hazards to humans and all living creatures. When you subtract the wasteful, you will gain and will be able to add up in what really counts, what really benefits your life, the lives of your loved ones, the life of the members of your community, the lives of all living things and our planet. It's a critical step in the right direction.

Living a greener life will not happen, until you learn to subtract and add. Subtract and add, a simple equation leading the world, and your life, your home, your bank account, and your peace of mind to a better place. When you start to subtract, you add to your life, happiness, financial freedom, freedom to have time to do what you like, and be able to choose to do so, all that will multiply.

"We do not inherit the earth from our ancestors, we borrow it from our children "~Native American Proverb

Think about how your everyday life is or isn't creating a better world for your children:

CHILDREN TURNING GREEN

Yes! This is the answer to the future. How many kids do I see as I walk the streets of NYC and see them carrying a disposable water bottle? So many of them take disposable utensils, napkins and snack bags in their lunch boxes. They are the future, and they learn by example. The school system is failing the world by not educating children in this regard.

Becoming a greener version of you is a lifestyle, a sum of actions that work to make the world a green, better place to live. Don't be silenced by society's way of interfering. We are responsible, as parents, to teach our children manners and good values, and how to live responsibly, with the good for all in mind.

Everything we do, our children observe and more often than not, will imitate. It is imperative, it is with most urgency, that we need to create consciousness within ourselves and for our children. Children learn from what we do. Do you buy bottled water as you go about your business? Or do you bring water from home in your own reusable bottle or recycled jar? Do you bring your own canvas shopping bags? Or do you follow that Swedish entrepreneur and just get a plastic bag with the 400 year life span? Do you make some of your own supplies? Do you buy bulk? What things do you do that your children will be do as well?

Besides doing and setting the example… do you share with them the reasons why making those choices is important? Do you talk to them about the lifespan of the plastic bags? Do you talk to them about why it's important to save water? My advice is that we should talk to them. Tell them what you think about the earth, show them what choices created big problems for our environment and why, and how they can be part of the solution.

Organize a park clean up, or a block clean up, so that they can better grasp the idea of trash, litter, waste, plastic, and the unnecessary wasteland we're turning the world into. Helping to clean up their block or their park can help create that consciousness which will lead to better choices, it will also help them understand how difficult it is to keep the world clean, one block at a time.

Take them places, take them to that composting event cities hold. Watch documentaries about the environment, about the world, about trash. Help them envision how tragic the idea of trash really is, but do so with a hopeful heart by pointing to the many options available and talk about people and organizations that are already working hard to be the change the world needs.

Talk about how their lunch box can contribute to change, using reusable water bottles, reusable utensils, reusable cloth napkins. Avoid plastic as much as possible.

If you do all that, and if you do all that consistently, you will slowly notice that your children will start making good choices all on their own, and teaching others about what they've learned all along.

My children and I organize a block clean up every year. We seldom have any helpers, but we still do it. We do it because it teaches them and it also teaches all the onlookers. It presents them with an opportunity to serve their community and set an example for others, connecting to the place where we live is important and helps create a sense of belonging; which according to research helps build self-esteem. You might wonder how do I start? How do I do something similar in my community? Well, when we hold our "It's My Block" clean up events, we post a sign two weeks in advance so that other neighbors and community members can consider the date and mark their calendars, we describe the activity and what will be made available to those who participate, such as: gloves and trash bags, we also ask that children be accompanied by an adult, and we describe the event as an opportunity to help clean the community clean. During the event we offer free lemonade to anyone who helps and brings their own reusable cup or mug. We clean up, pick up litter, and put trash where it belongs. We post signs about facts on plastic and pollution, and post a sign with some solutions we can all begin with as a first step. This provides an opportunity for children and their families learn and realize that they can make a difference in their communities and make them a cleaner and beautiful place to live. They can have create a direct impact in their communities, this creates a tremendous rewarding learning experience, and they have fun. They inspire each other and others.

Rituals:

Every time we are out and about, I created a ritual, I usually carry a reusable bag assigned as a trash bag, so as we walk through our city and we see a plastic bottle, or a fork, or paper plate, or empty bag of chips, or a plastic bag on the sidewalk, I pick it up, put it in our reusable trash bag, and dispose of the trash as soon as we see a city trash can. You may think that's not something you'd do, and I can understand that, because it's not nice to pick up other people's trash, but to me, it is a way of contributing, and educating my children not to litter, taking a step further by taking positive action about another person's inaction, to make our community a cleaner place. I recently read that there is a movement in Sweden, where people who jog carry a bag and pick up any litter that they encounter during their jogs. This is the same idea of what we've been doing for years, call it "strolling-ups?" Because as you stroll, or take your child for a walk on their stroller, you can help keep your city clean. It takes responsibility to teach your kids this idea of helping to keep a community clean and as green as possible, it's also important to teach them to always check in with you if they want to pick up trash, it must be okayed by an adult so they don't pick up anything that could harm them such as anything sharp or that is in a very filthy condition. I think that it may be easily assumed that it is obvious you must supervise them and offer gloves and antibacterial gel to protect and clean their little hands whenever they do this, but it is so gratifying to see their little faces smile knowing they helped in some way.

My children don't understand why people litter: that's the point!, everyone should think this way, and we'd have cleaner cities, rivers and oceans, but it does take a parent to teach them, and it does take that they see you not litter and it does take that they see you modeling the behavior you want to teach them. It's been years since we started the practice of picking up the trash we come along as we go about our daily lives, and to this day, years later, they take initiative to ask me if we could pick up the litter they see. It's no longer me pointing to the litter and explaining how we should pick it up, now it's them asking me to look in a certain direction so that I can see the trash in a given spot. They've acquired this practice, it's part of them now.

Was it always this way? Well, no, not really, it took all those strolls to the park and while running errands, and it took them seeing me clean up the trash laying around the park while they took their tennis lessons. We must all take responsibility of the rituals and customs we want our children to learn. If they see you littering, if they see you opening your car window and tossing a snack wrap, or if they see you toss your disposable coffee cup to the curb, they will eventually do the same. The same goes for the practice of using reusable cups and water bottles, cloth napkins, reusable grocery bags, etc.

"You must be the change you wish to see in the world "~Unknown

Think and make a list of the things you usually wish someone would do, then do at least one of those things:

BE INFORMED

Yes, because the chocolate bar you just bought at the store has a story behind it, do you know where chocolate comes from? How the people working to produce your chocolate bar live and what struggles and injustices they face? Do you know where the flowers you're buying for Valentine's Day come from and how getting them to your corner of the world impacted the world?   Are you aware of where the seafood you're about to cook came from and what waters it swam in before ending on your plate? Be informed, it's a responsibility, if you want to make better educated decisions, and such is or will be the case when your mind frame starts to realize that you can be a part of the solution to a greener world.

Read about sustainable lifestyles, look up organizations and learn about what they are working on and why.

Look up local organizations and participate of events they may offer, there are great learning opportunities and magnificent ways in which to benefit your community. For instance, the city of New York gave away one million trees between the years 2012 and 2015. All residents had to do was fill out an online form or call a local number to request trees planted at given addresses or intersections or their local parks. My family and I contributed by walking the streets of our neighborhood and writing down addresses, as well as intersections and requesting trees for those locations. Doing so was so gratifying because we saw many of the trees we had requested being planted right before our very eyes. Homes and intersections that had no trees now do, because we made the decision to make a difference, through a city program that enabled residents' power of action. So act, take a step, then another, influence your community in an empowering way. Talk to your councilman, ask what you can do to help.

Read about organizations that inform people on health hazards or environmental issues at hand, become involved whenever possible, even if it is just through social media, even it means writing a blog, talking to neighbors and friends, informing others. Some people are uninformed but as soon as they realize they too can make a difference, the learning experience can be a turning point for many, helping them to become more conscientious of their life choices, starting from that cup o' Joe in the morning, to the plastic bag they used to gladly accept from the cashier at the supermarket, to learning about the story behind the chocolate bar tucked away in their kitchen cupboard.

Being informed is crucial, we must know what is going on in our city, as well as other parts of the world, and how others live, how we change ecosystems because of the choices we make.

I am subscribed to several environmental pages and newsletters, some are informative of events and learning opportunities right here in NYC, some are informative on a state or national level, and many are publications created by international organizations, some from Costa Rica, Peru, Ecuador, the Amazon, Patagonia, some are about protecting ocean waters, some are about people making a difference in remote areas of the world, and those I find the most inspiring. There is a man in India, for instance, he lives in northeastern India, his name is *Jadav Payeng,* and he planted a forest, one tree at a time, today, the area his trees cover is approximately the size of Central Park in NYC. Can you imagine? One single man making such an incredible, selfless impact? This man is an inspiration. He should be mentioned in schools, and given recognition for his hard work, the kind of work that has as a result the selfless act of caring for our planet. After realizing the area where he lived needed help, as the floods were eroding the land, in 1979 he started single handedly planting seeds, he'd make holes and dig the seeds. He soon started seeing the trees he planted grow. He realized the biggest threat to his trees were other men. Still, he kept going and has been doing so for over thirty years.

Did he ever think "how can I be a difference maker if I can only plant a few seeds each day?" did the prospect of change over many years distract him and hold him back? No. He kept planting seeds, determined to make a positive impact on his environment.

This is the kind of role model we need. Reading about him with our children inspired us. Change can happen, change can seem intimidating, change can be unachievable. Results are seldom seen immediately. But such thoughts shouldn't deter us from still trying, still taking steps in the right direction. From planting a seed, to using a reusable coffee mug, and a canvas bag instead of a plastic bag, or giving cloth diapers a try, we can all contribute to a greater cause. Our project could lead to an immense change for the future. The world could be at a better place in thirty or fifty years if we all make a few changes, become more informed, let others inspire us, and we too, become role models.

Join my family and I, you won't be the only one making changes that can change the world. Think of Jadav Payeng whenever you doubt this. Another way of realizing how there are others working to be part of the solution for a better and environmentally friendly planet is to reach out to your community and any organizations they may network with so that you too can connect to others who are also working to make positive changes. There are communities that offer park clean ups, there are fairs and city events promoting tree planting or mulching events. Our city offered workshops to learn about composting and to learn how to install rain barrels. You could find out what your city offers and become involved.

Have you ever planted a tree? Have you ever planted a seed? Do so if you haven't. Contact your local councilman to request to volunteer at parks or city events involving tree planting events. Or simply plant a seed and see the magic of a plant grow. Make a plan for it:

WORLD ORGANIZATIONS

There are international organizations working for the greater good. They have professionals as well as volunteers working to protect the fragile ecosystems of the Amazon, such as is the case of a region in Peru known as the Andean Purna, Cloud Forest, and Lowland Rainforest. They hold educational programs for locals enabling them to learn about their environment, learn about a sustainable lifestyle, as well as inform them of the threats deforestation pose to their lives and the ecosystem. Such organizations work along with the local government and implement educational tools to be introduced during the high school years to help spread the word of the necessary steps to take to contribute to the health and survival of those very fragile and threatened areas.

It's my opinion, that every school system in the world should implement this as part of their studies. I know this is something we can't just do overnight, but it is a thought and an idea, and if the school system doesn't provide these learning opportunities then it is our responsibility as parents to educate our children about this important issue that affects forests, rivers, oceans, locals and the world as a whole. We're all responsible for the health of our planet. Countries around the world have implemented environmental awareness as part of their curriculum, some have blended some of the already established subjects with ecology and environmental studies. Some of the countries that have made it a point to include environmental education as part of their elementary and high school curriculum are Hong Kong, South Korea, Taiwan, Singapore. Others educate the public through parallel programs available at educational centers, such is the case of South Africa and India.*

Those countries have experienced high urban growth and with it, also greater levels of pollution and have managed to understand that education is key to improve their environments. Enabling the help from their residents is key as well, so they provide ample opportunities for people to participate of educational events geared to environmental programs. The city of New York offers youth after school programs that connect school age children with the environment through taking care of trees, cleaning up river banks, restoring the habitats of oysters found in local waters. They also organize mulching events to care for street trees, and they have a wide arrange of programs available as learning opportunities.

I believe all schools should implement programs to help

shape how children sense their community and the environment so that all children have a chance to learn they can be part of a greener world. School systems that include environmental education would be a great influence to shape a better and cleaner world.

Take note of how many trash bags you dispose of each day for a week. How many recyclable and not, and what can you do to reduce that amount of trash:

STAYING GREEN FOR LIFE

That is the main goal! Becoming a green enthusiast and staying green. Once you realize that the world needs a 'green human race' which I like to think that stands not only as a more mindful and environmentally friendly human being, but also and equally as important as a an undivided, equal, humanity, you'll realize green can also be the new and only human kind. Green is a color we

To stay green, you need to take tiny throughout your life, incorporate the new and sustainable traditions into your daily routines. Make the holidays the most important time of the year to resonate and align with your environmental ideals. Be green during the times when the stores and the billion dollar industries want most for you not to be. Always be inquisitive about the reasons behind a certain tradition, look up facts, become an environmental advocate, even if it only comes down to watering the grass in your apartment building's courtyard or carrying your own water bottle. Even if it means to just participate of your local park's clean up, even if it just means switching to cloth napkins.

Make the little changes you feel comfortable with making. One step at a time.

Then go the extra mile and go out of your comfort zone, take it one step further, make a new change, tell a friend or a co-worker about it, make your own reusable shopping bags. Shop less, sleep and rest more, clean less, read more, take strolls by the park more often. Call your loved ones and spend time with them instead of going shopping. Spend time with your children. Learn a skill, keep making changes, read, take care of yourself, not through clothes and objects, but by living a life more aligned with what's real in your life, buy organic food, go out for walks, plan a trip, keep spreading the word about becoming part of a green solution. Keep making changes, questioning traditions that don't feel aligned with what you want in your life and ask why and why not? Think about what you think is most important to the health of our planet, and our fellow human beings.

Ponder on the idea of how you can make the changes you need in your life and this is just another step toward realizing that.

Ponder on the idea of making all the necessary changes in order to become better citizens of our planet.

Always think. Never litter. Drink water, save water, always save water. Think off grid, even if you live in the city, think about how you and your family can use less of all the services we are connected to. Think about how living in an urban area does not mean you are disconnected from nature, on the contrary, you are part of a generation living in cities that work to be environmentally friendly. What you do matters. Cities and city dwellers need nature in their lives. Trees make cities beautiful, renew the air we breathe making cities healthier, and they even raise real estate values!

Consider only buying local and second hand.

Learn to make your own toiletries, your own laundry detergent, and your own disinfectant cleaning supplies. Start buying bulk, unsubscribe from junk mailing lists, plant a tree, plant a seed and see the seed grow into a tree. Water your garden, speak words of peace to everyone you meet.

Be mindful of others and their beliefs.

Ride your bike whenever possible. Have your children ride their bikes, or scooters whenever possible. Take mass transit whenever possible, make it a habit. Make whenever possible a daily phrase that will become your everyday thing. Enjoy every moment, life is too short not to make the changes the world needs right now. The world needs more people wanting to make positive impacts on the environment.

And hey, if you're going to be green, just like me, I thank you for it, and I am so glad my efforts will not be the only ones. Becoming a greener person is for life. Taking small steps toward a greener world, seems to be the only option if we are going to help our planet.

What is it that pulls you away from making lifestyle changes? How can you be a leader to set an example of change in your community? You are a difference maker too! Make a plan for the changes you want to lead:

References:

Research of historical facts retrieved from Wikepedia, research on environmental facts retrieved from Tree Hugger, The Clean Air Council, Crees Foundation, One Million Trees, and online searches.
Inspirational quotes belong to the celebrities who said them, as mentioned next to each quotation, and were gathered through careful internet searchesand readings regarding the environment, nature, the world and self. *Quotes by: Dr. Seuss, Annie Leonard, Mahatma Ghandi, John Muir, Native American Proverbs, Robert Swan, William Morris, Khalil Ghilbran, Henry David Thoreau, Joseph Campbell, Jane Goodall, Jim Rohn, Vincent, Van-Gogh, and anonymous quotes.*

Other References used:

* *Urban Context, "Four Asian Tigers" by*   Geok Chin Ivy Tan, John Chi-Kin Lee, Tzuchau Chang, and Chankook Kim

* *Cities as Opportunities, by* Daniel Fonseca de Andrade, Soul Shava, and Sanskriti Menon

* "Advancing Urbanization" by *David Maddox, Harini Nagendra, Thomas Elmqvist, and Alex Russ*

Disclosure

Please note that this book was created doing research on historical facts about traditions and acquired social modern life routines. Quotes and information presented in this book belongs to those who are mentioned as owning the quotes and information retrieved and research are also mentioned and this book does not claim ownership to those references nor to the quotes included. This book was written to help others in their path to becoming more environmentally friendly and conscious about their lifestyle choices to find a path and guide to start their journey on their choice of helping to create a greener world. All suggestions written on this book are sole examples of the changes I have put into practice and they represent a journey that has worked for my family and I, written with a love for the planet, other fellow human beings, a love for diversity and respect. By purchasing and reading this book you agree and understand that this book is only a narrative of my personal experience that also provides some facts and information through research. This book is a guide and may only be considered as such.

All written materials as well as illustrations are copy righted material that may not be copied or reproduced without the publisher's consent.